UNDERSTANDING "SENILITY"

Golden Age Books
Perspectives on Aging

UNDERSTANDING "SENILITY"

A LAYPERSON'S GUIDE

Virginia Fraser
and Susan M. Thornton

PROMETHEUS BOOKS
Buffalo, New York

Published 1987 by Prometheus Books
700 East Amherst Street, Buffalo, New York 14215

Library of Congress Cataloging-in-Publication Data

Fraser, Virginia.
    Understanding "senility".

    (Golden age books)
    Bibliography: p.
    1. Alzheimer's disease—Popular works.
I. Thornton, Susan M. II. Title. III. Series.
[DNLM: 1. Alzheimer's Disease—popular works.
WM 220 F842u]
RC523.F74   1987   618.97'683   86-30662

    ISBN 978-0-87975-392-4

Dedication

To Ada Gould Hart, mother of Virginia Hart
Fraser, who sensitized us to the pain and the
courage it takes to live with Alzheimer's Disease

Preface

This booklet had its beginnings in 1977 when Alzheimer's Disease was still being called "senility" or "hardening of the arteries." It was developed in part through the experience one of the authors had with her mother, who had what we now know to be Alzheimer's Disease. In trying to understand the behavior, she was told by her physician, as many others had been, "What do you expect, your mother is eighty-four!"

Thus began an intensive search for answers. A conference was held at Loretto Heights College in Denver on what was then the term of choice, "organic brain syndrome." Interviews were done with families of mentally impaired older persons to attempt to learn more about the need for education and assistance to this group of persons. A group was formed called "Network for Special Elders," which ultimately became a prototype for the Alzheimer's support groups that exist today.

The first printing of this book was done in 1979 as an initial attempt to provide some information to persons desparate for a description of what they were facing. It was a pioneering effort. Since that time many excellent publications have been produced. We have listed some of these on the bibliography and resource pages.

Between the time this volume was last published (1982) and the present edition, an explosive growth in education about Alzheimer's Disease has taken place. So much attention is now being focused on the disease that care must be taken not to diagnose a treatable ailment as Alzheimer's. We hope that this book can serve as an introduction to the issues surrounding this serious health problem.

Virginia Fraser
Medical Care and Research Foundation
1565 Clarkson Street
Denver, Colorado 80218

Susan M. Thornton
474 W. Easter Avenue
Littleton, Colorado 80120

Contents

1

Defining "Senility"

For many years "senility" has been a hidden topic, little discussed and even less understood by laypersons. Until "senility" strikes one's own family, most are relieved not to have to address the issue.

The images of "senility" are varied. For some, "senility" is an elderly man on a park bench staring at his feet for hours. Others envision an elderly woman muttering loudly to herself on the street. Encountering such evidence of impaired mental capacity, many feel embarrassed or fearful, and turn to walk rapidly away.

What does "senility" mean to *you* personally? Do you believe that everyone who lives long enough will begin to behave in a bizarre manner? Do you ignore the problem because it is upsetting or because you think nothing can really be done to improve the lot of the "senile" elderly? Most laypersons would answer affirmatively to these misconceptions, and most would admit that fear is a common and pervasive response to the topic of "senility." Because fear is usually greatest when ignorance or misinformation prevails, this volume, in its small way, has been designed to offer additional understanding.

The following three paragraphs describing "senility" in medical terms have been provided for those who desire a somewhat technical understanding of the topic. This is the only technical portion of our discussion, so if you find it heavy going, please continue reading. At least you will understand why the word *senility* is so often put in quotation marks!

Senility is a term commonly used by laypersons to describe the general decline in memory, concentrating ability, and thought processes that are believed to accompany aging. Professionals working in the field of aging generally dislike the word *senility* because it is so imprecise and because it can be used to describe conditions that could be successfully treated if correctly diagnosed. "Senility," properly speaking, is not a medical diagnosis at all. Indeed, some professionals call the word a "wastebasket" or meaningless term.

Two somewhat more specific medical terms for "senility" are *senile dementia* or *organic brain syndrome*. However, since most "senility" is caused by Alzheimer's Disease (see below), we will refer in this book to that disease instead of "senility."

An extremely small number of persons diagnosed as being mentally frail have long-term alcoholism, syphilis, or Parkinson's Disease. However, the vast majority are affected by Alzheimer's Disease, which is characterized by the brain changes. Smaller percentages of individuals suffer from a hemorrhage in the brain or from arteriosclerosis (hardening of the arteries) of the brain. Physicians used to believe that hardening of the arteries was the major cause of "senility." Recent careful studies, however, have shown that this is not the case.

Basically, Alzheimer's Disease involves brain changes that include the tangling of filaments and tubules within nerve cell bodies (fibrillary tangles), the deposition of certain carbohydrate substances outside nerve cells (senile plaques), and the appearance of small granules and vocules within nerve cells. The nerve cells that are being destroyed are the working components of the brain. They contain memories, receive and sort out sights and sounds from the environment, and send out the impulses to set muscles in motion. Nerve tissue affected by tangles and plaques looks dead.

There are two conditions that may appear similar to Alzheimer's Disease and can be confusing to the casual observer: the first is *delerium* and the second, *dementia*. Both can result in symptoms of mental impairment, confusion, or memory loss. Delirium can be caused by an illness or a reaction to medication, but with dementia there is an actual impairment in intellectual functioning. While dementia can be caused by a number of different diseases, such as stroke or thyroid malfunction, Alzheimer's Disease is the most frequent cause of irreversible impairment.

While the precise cause of Alzheimer's Disease is not yet known, much promising research is being conducted. Medical knowledge is changing almost daily, and there is hope that ways to prevent and effectively treat this difficult disease may yet be found.

2

Some Statistics

The size of the Alzheimer's Disease problem is large—and growing, because the number of older persons in America is increasing. More and more, dementia is being seen as one of the most significant public health issues of this century. Approximately two to three million Americans suffer some form of dementia, including over fifty percent of nursing home residents.

The prevalence of mental impairment increases with age from approximately three percent of those sixty-five to seventy-nine to more than twenty percent of those individuals who are eighty or more years old. The over-sixty-five population in the United States now totals eleven percent of the current 230 million population; this group is expected to increase to fifteen percent in the next fifteen years. In that same period, the over-eighty-five category will increase by fifty percent. Hence, it is likely that the absolute numbers of elders with Alzheimer's Disease will increase significantly in the next several decades.

3

Early Symptoms

The first symptom of Alzheimer's Disease that family members notice is an elder's loss of short-term or recent memory. The older person may be able to remember well an incident that occurred fifty years ago, but may forget the names of grandchildren or that a kettle has been left boiling on the stove. Typically, the person with Alzheimer's Disease may be forgetful about appointments, may seem to lose interest in his or her job or in hobbies, and may appear to be depressed. Some are very skillful at covering up this difficulty and denying that anything is wrong, while others suffer great frustration. Many times early symptoms are not recognized. Some individuals show a dramatic change in personality.

They may become irritable and easily upset, fearful or depressed; others simply withdraw.

Many persons with Alzheimer's lose a degree of what physicians call "cognitive ability": they become unable to think problems through logically to adequate conclusions. Difficulties may be experienced in balancing a checkbook or managing figures. While an elder may find it simple to cut up lettuce, slice tomatoes, and peel onions as separate tasks, when asked simply to make a salad without specific, step-by-step instructions, he or she may fail.

Next, confusion generally becomes quite noticeable, with the elder becoming confused about time and sometimes about place. Occasionally the person may even become lost in familiar surroundings. Concentration and reading ability are affected. There is increased difficulty with one's ability to screen out disturbing stimuli. The person may have difficulty making plans and may thus become easily frustrated.

It is important to note here that there is no typical pattern for the Alzheimer's patient. Indeed, inconsistency is normal. No single symptom or behavior, except for recent memory loss, is completely predictable. After weeks of failing to recognize a family member, suddenly the person is acknowledged. After days of garbled language, speech patterns become lucid. After months of not remembering places, recognition is there. At one moment an Alzheimer's victim may seem lucid, only to become totally confused an hour later. Although medical science has added greatly to our knowledge of the workings of the brain, much remains unknown.

Behavior may occur that is not thought by others to be appropriate. The person may take someone else's possessions, may dress and undress publicly, may make inappropriate comments. There is increasing difficulty in handling complex social situations. Difficult chores and hobbies are often abandoned.

It is at this point that families frequently find it impossible to relate to the individual in the same manner. Now the "child" begins to "parent" the parent, a role change that can be very distressful. Suddenly the parent who has been depended on and listened to becomes unable to care for him- or herself, unable to make decisions, unable to complete some of the most basic tasks of everyday life.

4

Later Behavior Patterns

Distortion of long-term memory begins to emerge with the older person being unable to remember many events in the distant past that earlier had been so clear. Prior to this time the family probably has been upset by the person's behavior; now, with long-term memory slipping away, the Alzheimer's patient will also become very aware of his or her condition. Frequently, when this awareness dawns, the person will become quite upset, agitated, or depressed.

The agitated person may be restless, anxious, or hyperactive. Some may seem unable to remain still. One older person may be intent on leaving a care facility to return home, even though home is hundreds of miles away. Another may pick incessantly at clothing or a pillow, or may constantly rearrange belongings. A third may be unable to sleep at night and thus wander about, risking a fall.

Commonly, these persons show signs of paranoia, believing that they are being persecuted. Other Alzheimer's victims seem driven to search for something they think is missing. Some may lose their memory of "good manners" and accuse family members or others of stealing clothing, household items, money, valued possessions, and the like.

It is hard to know just what is going through someone's head as they search fruitlessly for something familiar, a particular lost object, but it's important to remember that persons who have lost both past and recent memory and are unable to reason logically may naturally assume that a misplaced item has been stolen. A decline in hearing, eyesight, smell, and/or taste may add to feelings of paranoia. At this stage many with Alzheimer's Disease become substantially depressed because they are now realizing ever more clearly their loss of abilities.

With the decline of judgment may come a breakdown in social inhibitions. Some older persons, for example, may no longer be aware of taboos against undressing in public or engaging in normally private activities in the presence of others. Family members and care providers, who may be shocked by such occurrences, should remember that these manifestations are not a deliberate breach of protocol—rather they are the result of mental confusion and a loss of awareness of what is and is not considered appropriate.

As the disease progresses, many patients lose more and more ability to care for themselves. They may experience incontinence, an inability to feed themselves, or even an inability to walk. As was previously mentioned, many reach a nearly total vegetative state.

Just as there are wide differences among all individuals, there are tremendous variations in the manifestations of Alzheimer's Disease. Some mentally frail elders will show one symptom before another, and the intensity of various stages will vary from one individual to the next. In some elders, Alzheimer's Disease progresses quite swiftly, while in others it may be very slow. In short, there is simply no way of knowing precisely what will come next or how long any given stage will last.

5

Medical Care

It is distressing but true that if an individual really has Alzheimer's Disease, there is very little that modern science can
do directly to affect the progress or course of the disorder.
Certainly there is no cure—and once the condition sets in, it
will continue to progress. Sometimes, *careful* use of medications can ease the symptoms of those who are agitated, wandering, depressed, or paranoid. An extra caution here is that,
all too often, agitated behavior is inappropriately suppressed
by an overdose of medication. All medications should be
monitored carefully and regularly.

In addition, mentally frail elders can be stimulated to
remain as alert and involved as possible within the main-

stream of life. Physicians can monitor the person to make sure that physical conditions do not add to the problems of Alzheimer's Disease. In short, emphasis can be placed on maintaining the quality of life for the person, a right to which each of us is entitled at any age.

The correct diagnosis of Alzheimer's Disease is all-important. There are older people with symptoms of intellectual failure who actually have physical problems that can be treated and improved. Some doctors estimate that as many as thirty percent of those who could be diagnosed as "senile" may actually have a physical problem that can be corrected or at least mitigated, causing an improvement in mental status.

6

Diagnosing Alzheimer's Disease

When laypersons see an elder acting disoriented, they often make the assumption that he or she is "senile." However, there are many conditions that look like Alzheimer's Disease, but are in reality treatable. A thorough general physical examination (with special attention to neurologic and psychiatric factors) is essential to rule out physical causes before anyone is diagnosed as having the disease.

There are a number of conditions, such as stroke and depression, that can result in confusion and disorientation in the elderly, thus leading to an incorrect diagnosis of "senility." These might include the reaction to an anesthetic from a recent operation or to a change of environment (for example, entering a hospital or a nursing home). Dehydration can cause a similar response, as can an improper diet. Long-term causes that are treatable include an improperly functioning thyroid, a vitamin deficiency such as that leading to a condition called pellagra (niacin deficiency), and diabetes. Even an unrecognized hearing impairment can cause an older person to be labeled "senile" when in fact deafness has caused simple misunderstanding.

Few laypersons realize that elders cannot tolerate the same drug dosages as younger people. Both improper drug dosages and combinations of drugs can cause confusion and disorientation, and are major causes of the erroneous diagnosis of "senility." Drugs that affect the brain are especially likely to make the symptoms of mental impairment worse; these include barbiturates, sleeping pills, sedatives, and tranquilizers. In minor doses, some of these drugs may be helpful to confused or disoriented patients; but in large doses, or in combination, they may aggravate symptoms.

Many doctors of geriatric medicine, confronted with a confused elderly person and suspecting drugs as the cause, will take the individual completely off all medications that are not absolutely essential. Often the confusion quickly clears up. Additional needed drugs may then be re-introduced very slowly and in extremely small doses.

Depression, which is common in the elderly, is another factor that can often be confused with Alzheimer's Disease. Faced with the death of a spouse, an adult child, or a friend; feeling the lack of meaningful contribution to society; frustrated by the body's growing weakness; fearing an uncertain future; perhaps living in poverty and often lonely and isolated; many older Americans might appear to have good reason to be depressed! Depression may be combated by a trained professional willing to discuss a patient's fears, by improving the person's living arrangement, or by the use of antidepressant drugs. (However, unless a well-trained professional has found that the elder is really depressed, an antidepressant may make the symptoms of confusion and disorientation even worse.) There are ways in which family and friends can help to combat depression. It is important to be realistic and to deal with the present; not to tell someone, for example, that everything will get better or that he or she should cheer up and get busy. Telling the person to get back to normal may only intensify the depression. There are ways of assisting a person, organizing his or her routine, and establishing a quiet atmosphere that are supportive. If there has been talk of suicide, the person should not be left alone. It is important to remind the elder that depression is usually cyclical and he or she will feel better eventually.

Depression coupled with Alzheimer's Disease can make an individual appear to be extremely "senile." When the depression is eliminated, often it becomes obvious that only a minor loss of brain function has truly occurred. It is not unusual, however, for persons who have suffered memory loss to become depressed as a result of their awareness of a failing memory.

If mental confusion occurs very suddenly in a normally healthy elder, or if extreme confusion suddenly appears in an older person who demonstrates only minimal brain dysfunction, geriatric physicians suspect physical causes. Laypersons should be aware of this fact: generally the onslaught of true Alzheimer's Disease occurs gradually over a period of time. If confusion begins very suddenly, a thorough evaluation of the problem is essential.

The first requirement for an accurate diagnosis of any person displaying mental confusion is a complete physical examination, including blood chemistry and other laboratory tests, the examination being conducted preferably by a physician experienced in the management of such problems. Later, a series of mental examinations, ranging from the simple to the more complex, may be administered by the doctor or by a psychiatrist or trained social worker. These tests are designed to determine the extent of possible brain damage and to distinguish between Alzheimer's Disease and depression. A physician can pose simple questions that determine how aware a patient is of the world around him or her. One test, called the Mental Status Questionnaire, includes such questions as: How old are you? What is the day today? What is this place? Who is the President of the United States?

Depressed persons can answer these questions correctly, even if slowly; persons with Alzheimer's Disease are far less able, depending upon the severity of their condition. Questions must be asked in a low-key, tactful way so that the person does not become either afraid or angry, since either reaction would damage the ability to respond. (It is important to note that sometimes elders cannot answer such questions because their environments do not provide them with orienting cues such as readable clocks, calendars, and so on. This lack of cues can occur both in institutions and in private homes.)

7

Personality and Heredity

Often the issue is raised as to whether certain types of individuals are more prone to Alzheimer's Disease than others.
Are those who have been dependent, isolated, or withdrawn
all their lives more likely to suffer from mental confusion in
later years? There is little evidence that personality type is
related to the incidence of Alzheimer's Disease.

There may be personality changes that lead a person to
overreact in certain situations. Rage, anger, and stubbornness
may be protective reactions to his or her inability to deal
with even the smallest changes in a situation. A mood swing
may be a reaction to unfamiliar surroundings, confusion
aroused by too many people, too complex a situation, or the

inability at and subsequent frustration with performing a simple task. Swearing, sobbing, and refusal to bathe or go to bed are reactions that can seem to have no apparent cause.

It is important to try to perceive what the person is feeling when the brain is not working properly. New experiences can become terrifying. A calm, consistent, reassuring response is needed. Activities and surroundings must be simplified and easily grasped. It is essential to take one's time and not to rush the person. Arguing or even reasoning logically in response to erratic anger is useless.

Families often ask if mental frailty is hereditary. There are indications in recent research of a ten to fifteen percent genetic disposition to contract Alzheimer's Disease in the general population. There are further indications that certain families may be more likely to have several members at risk. It is still difficult to pin down this issue because of the late onset of the disease.

Researchers have recently become aware of a close connection between Down's Syndrome and Alzheimer's Disease. It appears that a large percentage of those with Down's Syndrome develop Alzheimer's, provided they live past the age of thirty-five.

8

Dismissing a Stereotype

In years past, public disinterest in the promotion of research into the cause and cure of mental impairment in the elderly may have stemmed from the belief that all older persons will eventually develop mental confusion. This is simply not true. Many older persons live to a great age without losing any of their mental acuity.

Our culture, with its emphasis on youth, beauty, and physical fitness, has a condition that is often called geronto-phobia, or a fear of old persons. Not only do we fear old people and fear becoming old ourselves, we also devalue age. We buy into the media stereotype of the crabby old woman, we laugh at the elderly man chasing young nurses, and in so doing we refuse to believe that we will ever get old ourselves.

If you have shared the stereotype on aging, you probably are not involved with elderly persons. If you were, you would find that all older persons are not confused, depressed, or depressing. Most are vigorous, alert, and have a lifetime of experience to share.

Society fears aging, dying, physical disability, and any form of mental impairment. As a consequence, we have paid little or no attention to the major issues facing older persons. Only now with a growing awareness of the numbers of older people, is there concern (and it is mostly economic) for the public policy issues that this growing segment of the population represents.

Fortunately, with recent public recognition of the enormous problem of Alzheimer's Disease, there is some hope that adequate resources may be devoted to a search for the causes of this debilitating affliction, to support for the caregivers, and to developing creative ways of handling the day-to-day living environment of impaired persons.

There are few specific psychological therapies that have been successful with Alzheimer's Disease. Some years ago, many nursing homes used "reality therapy" as an attempt to orient the person to time, day, and place. It became clear, however, that no real learning was taking place and the more perceptive caretakers wondered why it would matter to the Alzheimer's patient whether it was Tuesday or Thursday.

One technique that seems to have some real measure of success if used by trained personnel is "Validation Therapy." Naomi Feil's book, referred to in the resource list, basically presents a communication method for tuning in to the concerns of the confused person in a way that gives emotional support for issues they are attempting to deal with.

9

The Person Affected:
Emotions and Dignity

Families often wonder if Alzheimer's Disease is emotionally painful for the affected person. This seems to vary from one individual to another. Some are aware of memory lapses or the inability to remember their own actions, and thus become very upset, frustrated, or frightened. Others appear to have no insight as to memory loss or changing behavior. As a general rule, with increasing "senility" comes lessened ability to know what is happening. Some people in extreme stages of Alzheimer's Disease appear quite happy and comfortable, seemingly unaware of their condition. Others remain agitated and depressed, leading one to wonder if they may simply be unable to communicate their anxiety and suffering.

Families frequently ask how they can comfort a distressed relative who has Alzheimer's Disease. Family members should first be aware that often affected persons do not express their fear directly. One person may express anxiety regarding a physical problem, which he or she may feel is more "acceptable" than being open about a mental problem. He or she may become irritable and demanding about minor details. Emotions are very often close to the surface, and some afflicted persons may cry or experience rage more easily than they formerly did.

Probably the most important starting place for helping to understand the reality of the situation is to know as much about the disease process as possible. Alzheimer's victims are not who they used to be. They cannot understand and respond logically. Security, comfort, closeness, stability, routine, and kindness are the key elements for assisting the confused person. The caregiver must also recognize his or her own feelings of anger, frustration, fear, and embarrassment. Only in this way can the interaction be positive. It is the quality of the time spent with the Alzheimer's patient that can help most. Caregivers can learn to recognize what a supportive environment is, and what interests and activities the affected person still enjoys.

When the impaired person strikes out in a rage accusing his or her spouse of being an impostor, neither logic nor anger will help. Distraction may, however. A loving and empathic response may. It is nearly impossible to determine what provokes the anger. It could be a reaction to some confusing situation, an unconscious fear, or an inability to communicate.

Wandering is a characteristic problem. One wonders if the person just gets lost or is searching for home, for a lost self. Does it express restlessness, boredom, or a need for activity? A caregiver can help by seeing that the person gets enough activity each day.

Many people, both young and old, believe that asking for help is a sign of weakness. Confronted with this attitude, a care provider could suggest that to ask for help is instead a sign of strength. To ask for support is not an act of dependence; it is assertive. Asking for help when help is needed is the wise, mature thing to do. (Families should remember this themselves, if they are reluctant to seek emotional support for their own distress!)

How can families help persons with Alzheimer's Disease maintain their dignity? As a general rule, care providers should expect as much from an individual as that person is able to give. For example, the older person should be involved in as many decisions about his or her future as possible. Care providers must be realistic about this decision-making process, because elders who feel threatened by having too many or too difficult choices may react by becoming anxious and confused.

It is very demoralizing for anyone to be discussed by others as if he or she were an inanimate object; yet this is a pattern many elders experience. Even patients with minimal brain dysfunction are often discussed by family or professionals as if they were not present. Any person so treated is justified in responding as many do—with depression, withdrawal, and/or anger.

Older persons who must be moved from their own familiar environment are often demoralized. Indeed, a move can sometimes result in disorientation that looks like "senility." Confronted with a bustling new environment, strange noises, and unfamiliar sights and smells, an elder may become confused. Care providers should be aware that this may occur.

Personnel at hospitals, nursing homes, and other care facilities are becoming increasingly aware that elders often seem more comfortable when surrounded by their own possessions. By permitting residents to bring with them some furniture, pictures, or other anchors to the past, such facilities are giving residents a degree of comfort and their own sense of identity.

10

A Therapeutic Environment

Whether the person afflicted with Alzheimer's is at home, in an assisted living situation, in day care, or in a nursing home, there are elements in the environment that can promote well-being. First, the person must be accepted for who he or she is in a nonjudgmental fashion. Second, the environment must be one in which the person is encouraged to function at the optimum level of his or her capabilities. Third, the staff must understand the disease process and what individual characteristics the person expresses.

The environment must be safe from hazards of falling, free of harmful objects, and secure from outside dangers. It should be structured so that there is familiarity with respect to where things are and when events happen. It should contain personal belongings and familiar items. There should be sensory stimulation available: things to feel and hold. There should be places for quiet times, for music, and for visiting. The color, texture, design, and sound within the environment should promote relaxation.

Adaptive devices should be available to facilitate independence as long as possible. An example here might be the use of dinner plates with an edge for easier manipulation of food, or the serving of convenient finger foods.

Staff or care providers are needed who can take time to communicate nonverbally.

A therapeutic environment is needed that focuses on individual strengths rather than disabilities.

11

Housing Alternatives

Options for the housing of mentally frail persons are quite limited, as anyone who has sought a suitable living situation for an individual with Alzheimer's Disease can testify. In the early stages of the disease, the person can often remain at home, first managing alone and later with support systems such as home health care agencies, home-delivered meal programs, and day care. It is generally better for individuals to remain in their own homes for as long as possible.

Is it best for an elder who can no longer live alone to stay with an adult son or daughter? Or is placement in some kind of care facility or nursing home better? There is no simple answer here. Certainly the wishes of the person should be considered as much as is possible, but those with Alzheimer's Disease are not always realistic in their preferences.

When should such an older person live with his or her children? If the family has the room, resources, and desire to take in the elder, and if his or her physical problems are not too severe, perhaps the affected relative can live with grown children. However, if the older person is demanding, unreasonable, sleepless, or a tremendous physical and emotional burden on the family, a nursing home or other care facility may be a better choice. Many families use a day care situation to keep a parent at home. Others use the help of a respite care program where it is available.

Often families are wracked with guilt when they decide to put a parent in a care facility, remembering dreary stereotypes and fearing such placement as a final gesture. However, there can be benefits. In many nursing homes and care facilities there are more activities than in familial settings where all or most members work and the elder is left alone for long periods of time. Socialization with others may be helpful in itself. Perhaps Validation Therapy will be beneficial; or the person may need closer medical supervision and assistance than the family can give. Certainly there is no easy solution, no blueprint that will apply to all families and all situations.

Families will continue to have to make painful, individualized decisions about the living arrangements for a person with Alzheimer's Disease. Judgments will not only have to be made about what is best for the person, but a careful examination will need to be made concerning what is best for the family. Later we will examine the emotional stresses suffered by relatives in such situations, and offer suggestions for relief.

12

Selecting a Care Facility

Everyone has heard horror stories about nursing homes. While there remain some substandard facilities in this country, there are also those that do the best job possible. Families may wish to examine as many facilities as possible to learn for themselves what is offered at each. One of the best ways to judge a care facility is to visit unannounced. Some obvious things to look for are cleanliness, both of the facility and of the residents; the quality of food served; whether residents are engaged in activities or just lining the walls. Is the facility's general atmosphere warm and friendly or cold and sterile? Talk with residents and their families for further information. Call your local or state ombudsman program for assistance and guidance.

Some experts urge that families visit not only during the day, but at night as well, since the night shift in a nursing home is usually the most lightly staffed and may be the most difficult. Often elders awaken confused and afraid in the night. Does the staff simply give such persons sleeping pills and tell them to go back to sleep? Or do they talk and work with them until they are calmed and relaxed?

Families should talk not only with administrators of nursing homes, but with other members of the staff as well. Generally, how caring is the staff? Do staff members seem genuinely to like the elders? Are individualized conversations common between residents and staff? Is there some depth to these conversations, or does the staff seem patronizing? Do the aides seem cheerful or dour? Conversation with aides may be most important of all, since they often have the most contact with elderly residents.

Family members who examine nursing home facilities might look at the home's rehabilitation programs and activities. Do the activities go beyond simple tasks such as cutting out paper dolls? Do programs from the outside come into the nursing home? Equally important, do nursing home activities take those persons who are mobile (ambulatory and semi-ambulatory) outside the home periodically?

Families should ask questions about costs, of course, and should especially investigate any unusual fees. These might include added costs for such services as hand-feeding, incontinence, special diets, laundry, supplies, and so on.

A major concern for critics of long-term care facilities has been the over-use of tranquilizing drugs. Instead of working with patients who are upset, agitated, or in any way difficult, some care facilities and physicians have been quick to sedate them, making life a daze for the residents but simpler for the staff. This problem—it is to be hoped—is easing, but families might talk with their physician, the medical director, or the administrator of the care facility about this issue.

Finally, whenever possible, the nursing home should be close enough for convenient family visits. It would be ideal if the facility were also near the elder's old neighborhood so that non-family friends could visit. Obviously, these two ideals may not always be realized.

There are nursing homes that have special units or wings for the care of Alzheimer's residents. It is important to know what kind of training the staff has had for handling difficult behavior problems. Is the unit really geared toward the Alzheimer's patient or is it just locked to prevent wandering? Is there adequate space for activities and for walking outside in the fresh air? Are there activities appropriate to the needs of the Alzheimer's resident? Does the staff know how to handle sudden emotional outbursts? Is the environment adapted to reduce safety risks? Does a family support group exist? How is incontinence dealt with? What are the administration's policies on restraints?

There are steps families can take to prepare a person with Alzheimer's Disease for the move into a nursing home or other care facility. They should discuss the move with the elder, explaining honestly why the change is necessary and what the facility will be like. The explanation may have to be offered over and over again, perhaps letting the individual weep or express rage. Families should be realistic and not raise false expectations. For example, never promise that the elder's stay will be brief when this is known to be untrue.

The person's dignity may be protected by letting him or her help decide which facility is to be preferred if this is possible. Mutual agreement can also be reached on how often the family will visit, and the planning of items to take. However, some affected persons may be unable or unwilling to help make these decisions. If it is feasible, perhaps a preparatory visit by the elder to the facility will make admission day less tiring and confusing.

Many older persons quite naturally react with anger to being removed from a familiar setting. Despite chastisement, the family should remain supportive and understanding. Depression and lethargy may be other responses to placement in a long-term care facility.

Since an individual's dignity often suffers with such placement, family members should attempt to point out ways in which the elder remains important to them, and should continue to ask for his or her advice with family problems when appropriate.

13

Visiting the Elder

Family and friends may avoid visiting a mentally frail person, becoming uncomfortable when it is no longer possible to carry on the "normal" conversations of the past. In such a situation, imagination and creativity can help find activities meaningful to visitor and elder alike. Outings that both may enjoy can include taking a walk, going for a drive, or getting an ice cream cone.

In a care facility or in the affected person's home, some enjoyable visits may come from looking at photographs, playing simple games, reading aloud, reflecting on past happy times, working together on a craft project, or even doing simple exercises. If an older person lives in a nursing home and cannot get out, visits can be made to another resident—thus encouraging relationships with others. Because it is important that an elder stay in touch with old friends, letter-writing can be both therapeutic and enjoyable.

One daughter has found that giving manicures to her mother and to other women in a nursing home satisfies everyone. Such an activity creates a comfortable atmosphere; conversations seem less inhibited, and holding hands can create a special warmth.

Perhaps an inexpensive tape recorder can be brought on a visit. An elder can be encouraged to recall experiences from the past; describe a favorite childhood room, game, or set of clothing; or simply record messages for the grandchildren. A tape recorder can be an invaluable aid to capturing family history. Often when short-term memory is gone, the long-term memory remains intact. The most meaningful kind of visits, as observed from the delight on residents' faces, are those of small children and pets. Just watching and touching these welcome visitors brings contact and comfort to a sometimes sterile environment. Music and songs are often recalled long after memory cannot be reached.

Again, here are things to remember if you are the visitor. Keep the scene and activities simple. Give any instructions one step at a time; do not get irritated if the same questions are asked over and over again; do not expect the person to remember or identify names or things; and do not argue. Maintain a sense of humor.

Many Alzheimer's victims in the middle and later stages of the disease develop problems with coordination and spatial relations. They may misjudge depth or distance so that walking or sitting can be dangerous, and they may need guidance. It is very common for people not to be able to figure out where their body is in relation to where they need to move.

14

Stresses on the Family

Coping with Alzheimer's Disease is, for the family of an afflicted person, a painful and difficult task that can lead to great emotional stress. Feelings of helplessness, anger, guilt, shame, and depression may be experienced; the family may come to believe that it is alone in these feelings. Rest assured, you are *not* alone.

Helplessness is a common reaction of laypersons to mental frailty in their families. Unable to understand what causes dysfunction of the brain and fearing what the future will bring, families often feel trapped and helpless. The helplessness may eventually turn to anger. A daughter, for example, may become irrationally angry with her father for acting strangely and for causing her distress. This is not a response most families would wish, but it is a very real human reaction to severe stress. Anger with an elder often turns to shame. How can one be angry with an older person who cannot help him- or herself? The daughter feels she should be compassionate instead of angry and resentful, but cannot—and should not—deny her feelings.

Guilt is a very prevalent response among families. Haunted by the "if only I hads," families often feel that some action on their part could have prevented the Alzheimer's Disease. "If only I had been more attentive, Dad wouldn't be like this," a son may say. Obviously such feelings of guilt, although very real, are not logical. Families must recognize that nothing they could have said or done would have kept an elder from developing the disease.

In addition, much guilt usually surrounds placement in a care facility. The elder, having been raised in an age when families cared for their own older relatives, may demand that the family care for him or her at home. Although a daughter may have found this care impossible, she often still feels that somehow she should have been able to give it.

Families commonly grieve for a member with Alzheimer's Disease even before death occurs. Although this may sound unusual, it's not. Throughout life people grieve for losses not directly related to death: loss of a job, a marriage, a child who is going to college, for example. Experiencing Alzheimer's Disease, many family members find themselves grieving for the loss of those qualities and characteristics of their loved one to which they had grown accustomed. They also grieve because they must now assume a new role in the family. Or they grieve when an elder is placed in a nursing home or other facility, usually seeing such placement as a symbolic last placement before death.

Sometimes the emotional strain is so great that family members react in unusual ways. One such response is denial: families may deny that their elder is mentally impaired, insisting in the face of all the evidence to the contrary that the parent is perfectly all right. Some families make up for their guilt by overvisiting the elder in a care facility, perhaps berating the staff over minor problems. Still others are so upset by the entire situation that they may avoid visiting the elder completely. These families probably would benefit from support and even professional assistance until they find their equilibrium once again.

Families should remember a number of important truths about the emotional turmoil they experience. First, family members must realize that they had nothing whatsoever to do with causing the Alzheimer's Disease. This is a disease of as-yet-unknown origin, and no amount of prevention, love, or consideration could have prevented it.

It is important to remember that much of the person's behavior is beyond his or her control, that he or she is unable to stop pacing the floor or yelling in rage. These types of behavior are the result of damage to the brain. It is hard to believe that someone is not able to remember simple tasks such as dressing, eating, going to the bathroom, and the like. It is clear, however, that as the brain damage progresses it affects nearly all bodily functions.

Because the afflicted person's abilities may fluctuate from day to day, it is hard for the caretaker to know what to expect. Some people with mental impairment have hallucinations. They may see objects that are not there or perceive people stealing things when no such event is actually taking place. They may believe that because a bed rail is up at night, they have been put in jail.

One of the most difficult problems caretakers encounter

is that of night wandering. This can be exhausting for the family of the person who cannot be left to explore the house safely, who may fall, turn on the stove, or go outside. There is a condition with Alzheimer's known as "sundown syndrome." This describes a characteristic of agitated behavior late in the day. Reduced stimulation in the evening hours may calm the person down.

Another difficult problem for the caretaker or the staff of nursing homes is that of inappropriate sexual behavior. It is not uncommon for Alzheimer's patients to expose themselves in public. Sometimes the brain damage results in frequent demands for sexual activity.

Speaking softly and trying to redirect the focus of the night wanderer or the older person's sexual behavior can help.

Often families are quick to grasp almost any theory or hope for a "cure" because they feel guilty or frightened and want the elder to get better. Families should—either alone or with a professional—look realistically at the situation, evaluating what is within their control and what is not. In other words, family members need to examine all options, measure the trade-offs involved, and identify the real limits of what they can do.

Sibling battles are common and often bitter when a parent has Alzheimer's Disease. The grown child, who is frequently responsible for care, sometimes becomes angry that other siblings are not sharing the burden. It is helpful if this is made an open issue, in which all members of the family are able to discuss their feelings. The person responsible for care should be given much credit by other family members, and all should share as much responsibility as possible. If this issue is not talked out, it has the potential to lead to bitter feelings for many years.

Some persons experiencing Alzheimer's Disease become unrealistically demanding. In such cases, families need to know that they have the right to put themselves first after all reasonable needs of the elder have been met. Families need not feel guilty for refusing to respond to unreasonable demands. They may need to be firm and set some limits in order to protect their own mental health.

If the elder and a grown child have had a poor relationship for years, it is unrealistic for the child to believe that the relationship will improve with the beginnings of Alzheimer's Disease. Sometimes families see mental impairment as the final, angry rejection by a parent. Of course this is not so, but all should be aware that they may feel this rejection.

Another stressful situation may involve the relationship between family members and the staff of long-term healthcare facilities. Some staff members react defensively if families mention problems. Instead of seeing the family as an integral part of the care system, these staffers view interaction as being time-consuming and troublesome. Issues that arise may be labeled as originating because of the family's "guilt."

Families, on the other hand, may be so anxious and distraught over the placement of a parent that their responses may be unreasonable. If such a situation occurs, both family members and care facility staff should examine their own motivations and attempt to improve the interactions. Strengthened communication can benefit the person, the family, and the staff.

Despite the stereotype of unloving families eager to shut their elder away in a care facility, the reality is that most families are very concerned and caring. They are going through an extremely difficult time when dealing with a mentally frail elder, and should be given full credit for both their feelings and their efforts. Anyone working with these families should give them as much recognition and acceptance as possible to ease their burden. Most important, families should attempt to understand their own feelings and emotions in this difficult time. They should be made aware that their feelings of anger, fear, frustration, embarrassment, and guilt are not unique. It is often comforting simply for families to know that they are not alone in having these feelings.

15

Family Support

The past few years have seen the growth of support groups nationwide designed to offer assistance for many of the difficulties that people face. Among the most effective of these is the network of groups that help the families of Alzheimer's victims. Such groups have organized under the auspices of the Alzheimer's Disease and Related Disorders Association (ADRDA). There are ADRDA chapters in most major cities, each sponsoring family support groups. These regular meetings provide a forum for information sharing, for listening, and for caring. Many services are available from the national association itself. ADRDA has developed education and training packages designed to meet the needs of healthcare professionals and family members. Their assistance ranges from research information to practical tips on how to deal with incontinence. Please refer to the bibliography and resource list at the end of this volume for the ADRDA's telephone number from which information can be obtained.

In an informal survey of families conducted in 1977 and 1978 to determine where they turned for support, it was found that family members reached out most often for emotional support to friends or others within the family. The results were quite mixed, with some reporting good support and others reporting very little. Perhaps the most consistently good results were reported by those who talked with others who had experienced Alzheimer's Disease in their own families.

While family members and friends offer good support, the care provider may need more help than these individuals can realistically provide. Unfortunately, many families believe there is a stigma attached to seeking professional help for their emotional problems. They see it as a sign of weakness—instead of the sign of strength that it is. It is often a great help for families simply to share their feelings with a trained professional, being reassured that they need not be ashamed of their emotions. To deny or suppress feelings is to make a difficult situation even harder.

Most of the families in our interviews reported that they had sought support from a physician. The physician is usually the first professional encountered by families with a mentally frail elder, and so it is usually to physicians that these families turn for psychological support. Some doctors are extremely sympathetic and well trained, and may be the ideal source for family support. Others do not wish to be involved in nonmedical problems, while still others may not have adequate information about community resources or

Alzheimer's Disease itself. If families encounter an unwillingness or inability to help in a physician, they may wish to find a physician with more knowledge in geriatric medicine.

Another source of support for families can be a member of the clergy. Some families find that a minister, priest, or rabbi will listen well, help the family members understand the intensity of an emotion, and offer suggestions as to how emotional stress can be lessened.

Psychologists and psychiatrists offer similar help for families; they can be located through hospitals, nursing homes, or even the Yellow Pages of the telephone book. Each county in the United States now has the services of a mental health center that includes such professionals on its staff; families should feel free to contact such a center and ask to be referred.

Another source of support can come from social workers, many of whom have an intimate knowledge of family situations. Some have special training in handling Alzheimer's Disease patients and their family problems. These professionals can assist in dealing with emotionally difficult nursing home placements. Many are on staff at mental health centers, nursing homes, and hospitals, and county departments of social services.

Ideally, nursing homes should also provide family counseling and support services. When a social worker is not on staff, some families find a friendly nurse to talk with at the facility, or an aide to assist them informally.

To reiterate, because it is so important: families should seek emotional support in what is, at best, an extremely painful and difficult situation. Family members should not attempt to deal with problems alone when they feel overwhelmed—they should seek help.

SOME MAXIMS FOR CAREGIVERS:

- Take one day at a time.

- You can't make someone else happy.

- There are some problems that you just can't solve.

- Remember, it's the disease, not the person.

- Educate yourself.

- Share the burden.

- Take care of yourself—take time for yourself.

- Laugh.

16

Present and Future Challenges

Carl Eisdorfer (see bibliography), in an address given at a national conference on Alzheimer's Disease, spoke of the need for a coherent national policy for "long-term caring." It has been said that the measure of a society is how it treats its older citizens. Will we measure up? It is projected that by the year 2030, there will be at least eight million people with Alzheimer's Disease and related disorders living in the United States.

The good news is that so much has been done since the late 1970s. Alzheimer's has become almost a common word at the breakfast table. Few people, except in jest, still call it "old-timer's disease." Many excellent books have been written, and numerous insightful portrayals have been done on television. Money is being dedicated for research, and a strong national organization has evolved. Alzheimer's Disease has received and continues to draw the attention of the federal government, and many states have also supported Alzheimer's projects. A movie star has now been affected, and a children's book is on the store shelves.

The essential challenge comes once more from Carl Eisdorfer in his book *The Loss of Self*:

> Alzheimer's Disease is a cruel disorder. However, no matter how devastating it is, the essential humanity of the "person turned patient" remains. As the disease progresses, there is little or no hope of recovery of memory, but people do not consist of memory alone. People have feelings, imagination, desires, drives, will, and moral being. It is in these realms that there are ways to touch patients and let them touch us.

This is the essence of the therapeutic environment described in an earlier chapter: a focus on individual well-being. Much remains to be done. Some of the big questions concern finding the cause, finding the cure, and finding the resources for care. We need to get quick assistance to the caregivers, especially psychological and financial support. Alzheimer's Disease must be covered by federal catastrophic illness insurance plans. It must be categorized as a *disease* and *not* as a psychological disorder. Standards must be established for nursing homes as they attempt to deal with an ever-growing number of Alzheimer's cases and related disorders. Assisted living facilities must be developed to house Alzheimer's victims who do not need twenty-four-hour nursing care. Continual training is needed for healthcare providers who are confronted with problems associated with

Alzheimer's patients and their families. Finally, informed citizens can make important changes happen. Working to improve conditions for the Alzheimer's patient is truly an investment in our own future.

Appendices

A. Results of Family Interviews

B. A Checklist for Alzheimer's Patients and Their Families

C. Some Thoughts on Moving to a Nursing Home

D. A "Sensual" Tour of a Nursing Home

E. A Consumers' Guide to Nursing Home Admission Agreements

F. A Consumer Perspective on Quality Care: The Resident's Point of View

G. Decision-making and the Mentally Impaired: Rights in Conflict

H. Federal Regulations on Patients' Rights

Appendix A

Results of Family Interviews

During late 1977 and early 1978 a series of interviews were conducted in the Denver, Colorado, area with families who were experiencing or who had experienced Alzheimer's Disease. The interviews were designed to provide background information for the first edition of this publication.

It must be emphasized that this study was not conducted along strictly scientific lines. The sampling of twenty interviews was too small to be statistically valid. Names of the persons interviewed were not selected at random, nor was consideration given to balancing age, sex, income, education, or other socioeconomic factors. The interviews were informal rather than structured; nevertheless, we believe the study reflects in general terms the kinds of problems and emotions experienced by many families.

CONDUCT OF THE INTERVIEWS

Twenty interviews were conducted in a period of approximately four months with twenty-one persons in regard to twenty-one elders identified by the families, physicians, or nursing home personnel as "senile." Of the twenty-one persons interviewed, seventeen were women and four were men, and all but three of these were (or had been) responsible for arranging care for the persons involved.

Of the twenty-one elders discussed, seventeen were women and four were men; seventeen were living and four were deceased.

AN INFORMAL METHODOLOGY

The results of the interviews were highly subjective. Although many of the families interviewed had experiences they did not relate for a variety of reasons, we recorded only those specifically mentioned during the course of the interviews. Some of the individuals interviewed were less than candid—for example, three denied completely that their elders were in any way mentally impaired.

The responses we obtained were those of laypersons, whose descriptions of early symptoms, medical problems, and indeed, their own actions, were doubtless skewed by their own fears, lack of information, and desire to appear in the best light.

Many of the figures mentioned below will not total the

twenty-one persons interviewed. This is because all mentions by families were recorded, and many expressed more than one symptom, emotion, etc.

CHARACTERISTICS OF THE ELDERS

Several of the persons interviewed believed that certain types of individuals are more likely to become "senile" than others—for example, that dependent individuals who center their lives around their families might be more prone than others to the condition in later years. Based on the interviews conducted and on information from medical experts, we found little evidence that any particular character type was more likely than another to become mentally frail.

Seven of the elders were described by their family members as having been dependent individuals throughout life, suffering feelings of inferiority and with few interests and friends. In contrast, five were described as having been bright, independent people with many interests and friends. Four were described as having been very emotional or "high strung" and three as having been domineering.

Four of the elders, all women, were described as having centered their lives around their families; two of the men were labeled as having been "workaholics."

And six of those interviewed mentioned that they had had a poor life-long relationship with the individual in question. How many others this might have been true of, although it was not admitted, is unknown.

EARLY SYMPTOMS

Symptoms marking the onslaught of mental confusion in later years similarly failed to fall into a clear pattern. The largest number (seventeen) of those interviewed mentioned incidents involving "loss of memory" during the early stages of mental frailty. Fourteen mentioned loss of mental acuity (nine specifically commenting on the increased difficulty the person had in managing dollar figures or playing numerical games). Eight mentioned changes in personality (including becoming "cranky" or argumentative), and another eight mentioned that the elder began to neglect his or her physical care, appearance and/or environment. Five mentioned loss of interest in the world and general withdrawal, five mentioned symptoms of insecurity, and four mentioned delusions or hallucinations.

EMOTIONAL RESPONSE OF THE FAMILIES

The emotions of those interviewed were often extremely painful and expressed by some only with difficulty. Doubtless not all of those interviewed described the full range of emotional difficulties with which they had dealt.

In the course of the interviews, emotions directly related to sorrow were mentioned fifteen times, with six of those interviewed crying as they described their experiences. Eight times fear was expressed, one for the future of their elder and seven for their own futures. Eight persons expressed emotions related to anger, five feelings of helplessness, four of guilt, and four a desire for the death of the elder. Three mentioned the physical hardship of managing their own lives while coping with the problems of a mentally frail relative, and one described the experience as a "nightmare." Three seemed to compensate for their feelings of guilt and past difficulties with the elder by seeking to "prove love" through such gestures as over-frequent visits to nursing homes.

Interestingly, two of those interviewed denied that their elders were in any way mentally impaired, although information from the physician and/or nursing home was strongly to the contrary.

DESCRIPTION OF PHYSICIANS' RESPONSES

Every person interviewed had interacted with a physician, both for medical care and assistance with the elder's declining mental acuity. The families all (with one exception, himself a physician) also turned to physicians for both information and for emotional support. It seems clear that whatever other emotional assistance families seek, either formally or informally, the physician is usually the first source of support to which families turn.

It is therefore unfortunate that of the twenty-one persons interviwed, most did not feel their physician had met their needs. Fully twenty expressed generally unfavorable comments about the physicians from whom they had sought emotional assistance. It must be noted, of course, that in this emotionally charged atmosphere the families may have placed unrealistic demands on the physician and that today most physicians are presumably better informed about families' feelings.

Seven of the twenty-one persons interviewed called the physician "indifferent" to their problems and the problems of the elder. Three complained that the physician refused to visit the nursing home—a source of considerable bitterness.

Three stated that the physician avoided talking with the family, three that he or she avoided talking with the person, and one that the physician seemed interested only in medical problems.

(It should be noted that these figures do not total twenty-one; some of those interviewed described experiences with more than one physician.)

OTHER SOURCES OF EMOTIONAL
SUPPORT FOR FAMILIES

If physicians generally did not meet the emotional needs of the persons interviewed, where did families seek or find emotional support?

Of those interviewed, turning to their immediate families for such support was mentioned thirty-seven times. Fourteen said they turned to their own spouses, and eleven to their own children. Results of such in-family support-seeking were mixed, with good support mentioned twenty-one of thirty-seven times, with average support mentioned four times, and with poor support mentioned twelve times.

Within the thirty-seven mentions of in-family support, siblings of the persons interviewed were mentioned eight times, with four of those results described as poor and only three as good. Siblings of the elder were mentioned four times, with three of those recorded as poor and only one as good. It should be noted that particular bitterness seemed to be involved when the sibling of either the person interviewed or of the elder failed to give good support.

Looking outside the family, eleven of those interviewed mentioned seeking emotional assistance from their friends (six with good and four with poor results). The most consistently good results in this area (four, all described as good) seemed to come from a friend who had experienced mental impairment of an elder in his or her own family.

Seeking emotional support from church-related sources was described only three times, but in each case it was reported as yielding good results. Another three persons said they sought help at the nursing home, with only one saying the response there was good and two saying it was average.

Only two of those interviewed described seeking professional help, but both results were rated good. It should be noted that some individuals may be reluctant to admit having sought this kind of assistance.

And significantly, three of those interviewed seemed to have turned entirely inward, either refusing to seek help from others or seeking it, and being rebuffed, having withdrawn completely.

Appendix B

Checklist for Alzheimer's Patients and Their Families

OBTAIN A THOROUGH DIAGNOSIS

    —Social and medical history
    —"Neuro-psychological" work-up
        including: —Face-hand test
                —Mental Status Questionnaire
                —Memory for Digits Test
                —CAT scan

PLAN A STRATEGY

    —Respite care

—Day care
—Information on nursing homes and their
          eligibility requirements
—Financial planning
—Decision-making plan
     —Power of Attorney
     —Durable Power of Attorney
     —Guardianship
     —Developing a Last Will and Testament
     —Developing a Living Will
     —Conservatorship

LOCATE AS MUCH INFORMATION AS POSSIBLE

1. On Alzheimer's Disease
    —Books and tapes
    —Tips for caregivers
    —ADRDA meetings in your area
    —Appropriate support groups in your area
2. On respite care and day care
3. On medical coverage
4. On insurance coverage
5. On support systems available to relieve families

Appendix C

Some Thoughts on Moving to a Nursing Home

Please don't call me guilty—I'm just scared

We're both alone together mother and I. Today, yesterday and many tomorrows, but especially today.

We're both scared in our aloneness, unable to comfort each other.

Mother—trying to be dignified in her terror of moving into the unknown.

My own unspeakable darkness of spirit—making this decision *for* her because she can't.

Because her mind is jumbled in her dignity.
Her manners are perfection and her mind is a mess.

Her scare is the fleeting awareness that she's lost herself, she
can't think who she is.

My scare is for us both—I'm scared that she trusts me—can
she? Should she? How can *I* be *her* self?

We move her into a space of less than 35 square feet, she
who loves the out of doors, a roommate too—she wouldn't
even share a motel room with her best friend because she
snored.

We bring her Hummel figure, a throw, some bells—My God,
when my baby was two and had the croup, I took her
favorite blanket to the hospital.

If I had a brother or sister would the pain be this intense?

How can I leave my mother in this unknown camp? Subject
her to the possible ridicule of others who don't understand
who she is.

Because now her self is hidden so far inside and the outside
looks so scattery and strange, and they won't know her.

Mother, please help me.
I'm so alone and scared.

Virginia Fraser

Appendix D

A "Sensual" Tour
of a Nursing Home

SIGHT

—Are staff interacting positively with residents? Are they smiling or do they look harried and hurried?

—Are residents clean and neat (e.g., nails clean, hair combed, proper clothing)?

—Do rooms have personal belongings?

—Is food attractively served?

—Are doorways, obstructions, etc., clearly marked for the visually impaired?

—Is lighting adequate?

—Are calendars large and hung low?

—Is the facility attractively decorated? Is it clean?

—Are the windows accessible and clean?

—Are the grounds and porches well kept? Are they used by residents?

—Is the furniture in good shape and appropriate?

—Does the staff show genuine interest and are they caring?

—Are pets utilized?

—Where do staff spend most of their time?

—How are stairways and doors protected?

—Are residents left in chairs for long periods?

—Are wheelchair residents walked?

—Are nurses on the floor or only at the desk?

—Do residents feel free to voice concerns?

—Is there a resident council? If so, are its meetings run by the residents?

—Are social services provided by a trained social worker?

—Does the administrator know residents' names?

—Is there a family council?

SOUND

—Is the intercom used excessively?

—What tone of voice is used to communicate with residents?

—Is there excessive noise?

—Are call-bells answered promptly?

—How are residents made aware of activities?

TASTE

—Observe mealtimes. Are portions adequate? Are there alternate selections? What snacks are available between meals? How are residents who require assistance during meals dealt with?

—Is water or juice available at meals and between meals?

—Do residents have the opportunity to have a special meal of the month where they plan the menu?

SMELL

—Do foul odors pervade?

—Are rooms well ventilated?

—How is incontinence handled?

—Are bathrooms clean and free from odor?

—Are residents free from unpleasant odors?

TOUCH

—Does the staff use touch in communicating with residents?

—Are room temperatures appropriate?

—Does the skin of residents feel well hydrated and not excessively dry?

Appendix E

A Consumers' Guide to Nursing Home Admission Agreements*

WHAT IS AN ADMISSION AGREEMENT AND WHY IS IT IMPORTANT?

An admission agreement is a legal contract between the nursing home and resident (or person who is legally responsible for the resident). Most admission agreements are written in "legalese," and are hard to understand. Because these agreements are legal documents, it's very important for you to *read and understand* what you are signing. The following

---

*From the office of Colorado's Long-Term Care Ombudsman.

brief guidelines are to help you better understand admission agreements. In addition, you might consider having a lawyer review the agreement with you.

ADMISSION AND DISCHARGE

Under federal law, a nursing home cannot require a person receiving Medicaid to pay higher "private pay" rates for a period of time, cannot require Medicaid residents to pay a "deposit" to be admitted, and cannot discharge a resident who changes from "private pay" to Medicaid. If you find one of these clauses in an admission agreement, call the Long-Term Care Ombudsman's office in your state.

Federal law states that a nursing home resident may only be discharged for medical reasons, the resident's welfare or the welfare of other residents, or for nonpayment for services. Beware of an admission agreement that says the facility can discharge a resident at its discretion.

Be sure the agreement spells out the nursing home's policy regarding a bed for a resident who is transferred to a hospital. Residents usually have to pay to have their bed held. Medicaid does not cover such charges.

PERSONAL AND MEDICAL SERVICES

The admission agreement should be specific about the kinds of services the home will provide (such as medical and nursing services, physical therapy, and so on). It should also spell out which services are included in the base fee—and which will cost extra.

The nursing home cannot legally bill a Medicaid resident for services covered by Medicaid. Medicaid residents who are receiving additional bills should ask the nursing home and/or their state Ombudsman's Program what Medicaid covers to make sure the monthly statement is accurate.

MEDICAL TREATMENT

Most admission agreements require the resident to comply with a doctor's orders. However, state and federal law give residents the right to refuse treatment, and a resident cannot be discharged for exercising this right.

PHARMACY SERVICES

The admission agreement should state that the resident can choose his or her own pharmacy. If a resident uses his or her own pharmacy, the admission agreement may require that the pharmacy package the resident's medications in the dosage system used by the facility.

DENTAL SERVICES

Some admission agreements state that participation in a dental check-up program is required. However, if you don't want to participate, you have the right to have this provision crossed out of the agreement.

PRIVACY

Under federal law, no medical or personal records can be released without the resident's permission. (There are a few exceptions, in the case of Medicare, Medicaid, and private health insurance companies.)

Some admission agreements ask for permission to take pictures of or to tape record residents. If you do not want to agree, have this marked out on the agreement, and both you and the admissions personnel should initial it.

FINANCIAL STATEMENTS

This is a very important part of the admission agreement, so *stop and read it before you sign.*

Most agreements state that the resident will be charged for late payments. However, if the resident receives Medicaid, this should be crossed out of the agreement and initialed by the resident and admissions personnel.

Anyone who signs as a "responsible party" or "guarantor" becomes responsible for all the resident's financial obligations. It's just like co-signing a loan for someone else. If the resident receives Medicaid, the home cannot require that the resident must have a "guarantor" to be admitted.

WAIVERS OF LIABILITY

Many admission agreements state that the home is not responsible for any loss or damage to residents' property. However, federally-developed residents' rights state that a nursing home must provide a secure place for personal property. Even if the agreement you sign states that the home is not responsible, if you have a major loss, you should ask about replacement and perhaps consider contacting a legal advocate if you receive no satisfaction.

TERMINATION OF THE AGREEMENT

The admission agreement should specify how the agreement can be terminated by either the home or the resident. Medicaid residents should not be required to pay a penalty for not giving advanced notice of discharge, and requiring the approval of a physician before the resident is discharged is a violation of the resident's right to refuse medical treatment.

Appendix F

A Consumer Perspective on Quality Care: The Resident's Point of View

This national research project was developed by the National Citizens' Coalition for Nursing Home Reform in order to determine residents' views on what makes life in a nursing home good, what is quality care, and what can be done to achieve it. Prior to this study, no research existed in which residents themselves were asked to give their opinions and to describe what constitutes good care in their eyes. Discussions were held with over four-hundred residents representing about seventy nursing homes nationwide. Their thoughts were recorded and analyzed for content related to quality care issues.

The following statements were mentioned most frequently:

Staff—good attitudes and feelings, prompt attention to needs, good care by staff, adequate number of staff, qualified staff, selection and training, continuity, staff supervision.

Environmental—private rooms, larger rooms, security, temperature controls, privacy, quiet, call light visible and responded to.

Food—variety, choices, proper preparation, served hot, pleasant and proper service, evening snacks, resident input, "home-style cooking."

Activities—variety, social activities, games, field trips, outings, eating in restaurants, arts and crafts, activities that "use your mind," community involvement.

Medical Care—physicians responding promptly, opportunity to see physician privately, ability to communicate.

Cleanliness—facility in general, particularly bathrooms, staff, food preparation sanitation.

Administration—good strong administration, supervision by administration, enforcement of rules.

Religion.

Resident council, residents' rights, participation in community activities.

Transportation.

Choices—regarding food, activities, decisions, doctors, roommates, bathing, bedtime, personal care staff.

Problem Resolution—resident councils, social workers, timely response from administration, appropriate staff, suggestion box, grievance committee, participation by advocates and families.

Quality-of-Life—choices, food, more and better staff, visitors, independence, more baths, less "hurry up and wait," compatible roommates.

Appendix G

Decision-making and the Mentally Impaired: Rights in Conflict

What is the implication for residents' rights when a resident is no longer able to make decisions yet hasn't been legally declared incompetent?

What happens when a resident's right to make choices is in conflict with the right to good medical treatment? What is the least restrictive alternative for the wandering combative person with Alzheimer's Disease who refuses to eat? What happens when a resident who cannot express his or her wishes continually pulls out the feeding tube? What about the resident who is terminally ill, and one member of the family insists on hospitalization? How about the resident who takes another resident's possessions? Who makes the decisions, whose rights prevail? The problems look like this:

- freedom from confinement versus safety
- choice versus substitute decision-making
- freedom versus restraint
- one roommate's right versus another's
- adequate nutrition versus refusal to eat
- choice versus need for medication

It is estimated that fifty to sixty percent of long-term care residents have some mental impairment. Very few have been legally adjudicated and have substitute decision-makers. In many cases the family may assume that they have the ultimate right to make decisions.

There are no clear answers and little definitive work has been written. The American Health Care Association does have a booklet titled *Questionably Competent Long Term Care Residents—Problems and Possible Solutions* that may help those who have questions.

Currently the focus of many questions involves right to die procedures, the ethical questions about when to pull the plug. For the most part, the current state of the art is that decisions tend to be made in an informal manner. There is increasing concern, however, that the rights of residents may not be protected or that their individual dignity may not be respected.

The care provider may be caught in a conflict of duty and liability. Given the current litigious nature of our society, many persons may look toward guardianship as the answer. This approach could conceivably backlog the courts and take away civil liberties unnecessarily.

While there are few definitive answers, here are some approaches to be considered:

1. How can the dignity and prior wishes of the individual best be respected?

2. Has the staff been sensitized to ethical dilemmas?

3. Have a variety of options been examined?

4. Does the nursing home have policies that help? Are these policies spelled out to families, residents, and staff?

5. Is there a durable power of attorney or a living will?

6. Can an interdisciplinary care planning process assist in objective decision-making?

7. Is there sensitivity and education about dying for the residents, family, and staff?

8. Is the staff trained in dealing with behavior problems, avoiding resistant areas with Alzheimer's patients?

9. Are issues thoroughly documented?

10. Would an ethics committee help?

11. Can the state Ombudsman help?

12. Is adult protective services intervention warranted?

A resident may not be able to act on all these rights. He or she may no longer be able to handle financial affairs, choose which dress to wear, participate in the resident council, or participate in planning medical treatment. But other rights are paramount—"the right to be treated courteously, fairly, and with the fullest measure of dignity," to receive adequate and appropriate health care.

Appendix H

Federal Regulations
on Patients' Rights

CHAPTER IV—HEALTH CARE FINANCING ADMINISTRATION
§ 405.1121

Title 42—Public Health

(k) *Standard: Patients' Rights.* The governing body of the facility establishes written policies regarding the rights and responsibilities of patients and, through the administrator, is responsible for development of, and adherence to, procedures implementing such policies. These policies and procedures are made available to patients, to any guardians, next of kin, sponsoring agency(ies), or representative payees selected pursuant to section 205 (j) of the Social Security Act, and Subpart Q of 20 CFR Part 404, and to the public. The staff of the facility is trained and involved in the implementation of these policies and procedures. These patients' rights policies and procedures ensure that, at least, each patient admitted to the facility:

(1) Is fully informed, as evidenced by the patient's written acknowledgment, prior to or at the time of admission and during stay, of these rights and of all rules and regulations governing patient conduct and responsibilities;

(2) Is fully informed, prior to or at the time of admission and during stay, of services available in the facility, and of related charges including any charges for services not covered under titles XVIII or XIX of the Social Security Act, or not covered by the facility's basic per diem rate;

(3) Is fully informed, by a physician, of his medical condition unless medically contraindicated (as documented, by a physician, in his medical record), and is afforded the opportunity to participate in the planning of his medical treatment and to refuse to participate in experimental research;

(4) Is transferred or discharged only for medical reasons, or for his welfare or that of other patients, or for nonpayment of his stay (except as prohibited by titles XVIII or XIX of the Social Security Act), and is given reasonable advance notice to ensure orderly transfer or discharge, and such actions are documented in his medical record;

(5) Is encouraged and assisted, throughout his period of stay, to exercise his rights as a patient and as a citizen, and to this end may voice grievances and recommend changes in policies and services to facility staff and/or to outside representatives of his choice, free from restraint, interference, coercion, discrimination, or reprisal;

(6) May manage his personal financial affairs, or is given at least a quarterly accounting of financial transactions made on his behalf should the facility accept his written delegation of this responsibility to the facility for any period of time in conformance with State law;

(7) Is free from mental and physical abuse, and free from chemical and (except in emergencies) physical restraints except as authorized in writing by a physician for a specified and limited period of time, or when necessary to protect the patient from injury to himself or to others;

(8) Is assured confidential treatment of his personal and medical records, and may approve or refuse their release to any individual outside the facility, except, in case of his transfer to another health care institution, or as required by law or third-party payment contract;

(9) Is treated with consideration, respect, and full recognition of his dignity and individuality, including privacy in treatment and in care for his personal needs;

(10) Is not required to perform services for the facility that are not included for therapeutic purposes in his plan of care;

(11) May associate and communicate privately with persons of his choice, and send and receive his personal mail unopened, unless medically contraindicated (as documented by his physician in his medical record);

(12) May meet with, and participate in activities of, social, religious, and community groups at his discretion, unless medically contraindicated (as documented by his physician in his medical record);

(13) May retain and use his personal clothing and possessions as space permits, unless to do so would infringe upon rights of other patients, and unless medically contraindicated (as documented by his physician in his medical record); and

(14) If married, is assured privacy for visits by his/her spouse; if both are inpatients in the facility, they are permitted to share a room, unless medically contraindicated (as documented by the attending physician in the medical record).

All rights and responsibilities specified in paragraphs (k) (1) through (4) of this section—as they pertain to (i) a patient adjudicated incompetent in accordance with State law, (ii) a patient who is found, by his physician, to be medically incapable of understanding these rights, or (iii) a patient who exhibits a communication barrier—devolve to such patient's guardian, next of kin, sponsoring agency(ies), or representative payee (except when the facility itself is representative payee) selected pursuant to section 205(j) of the Social Security Act and Subpart Q of 20 CFR Part 404.

Bibliography and Resource List

PUBLICATIONS

Bennett, Clifford. *Nursing Home Life: What It Is and What It Could Be*. New York: Tiresias Press, Inc., 1980.

Burger, Sarah Greene and Martha D'Erasmo. *Living in a Nursing Home: A Complete Guide for Residents, Their Families, and Friends*. New York: Seabury Press, 1976.

Cohen, Donna and Carl Eisdorfer. *The Loss of Self*. New York: W. W. Norton, 1986.

Feil, Naomi. *Validation Therapy, The Feil Method: How to Help the Disoriented Old-Old*. Cleveland, Ohio: Edward Feil Productions, 1982.

Guthrie, Donna. *Grandpa Doesn't Know Me.* New York: Human Sciences Press, 1986.

Gwyther, Lisa. *Care of Alzheimer's Patients: A Manual for Nursing Home Staff.* Chicago, Ill.: American Health Care Association and the Alzheimer's Disease and Related Disorders Association, 1985.

Heston, Leonard and June White. *Dementia: A Practical Guide to Alzheimer's Disease and Related Illnesses.* New York: W. H. Freeman, 1983.

Karr, Katherine. *What Do I Do, How to Care for, Comfort, and Commune with Your Nursing Home Elder.* New York: Haworth Press, 1985.

Mace, Nancy and Peter Rabins. *The 36-Hour Day: A Family Guide to Caring for Persons with Alzheimer's Disease, Relating Dementing Illness and Memory Loss in Later Life.* Baltimore, Md.: The Johns Hopkins University Press, 1981.

Otten, Jane and Florence Shelley. *When Your Parents Grow Old.* New York: Signet Books, New American Library, 1977.

Powell, Lenore and Katie Courtice. *Alzheimer's Disease: A Guide for Families.* Reading, Mass.: Addison-Wesley, 1986.

Richards, Marty et al. *Choosing a Nursing Home: A Guide for Families.* Seattle, Wash.: University of Washington Press, 1985.

Schwartz, Arthur D. *Survival Handbook for Children of Aging Parents.* Chicago: Follett Publishing Co., 1977.

Silverstone, Barbara and Helen Kandell Hyman. *You and Your Aging Parent.* New York: Pantheon Books, 1976.

OFFICES AND ORGANIZATIONS

Alzheimer's Disease and Related Disorders Association
70 East Lake Street
Chicago, Illinois 60601
Phone 1-800-621-0379 (Illinois Residents: 1-800-572-6037)

OMBUDSMAN PROGRAMS

Each state has a long-term care ombudsman program that can be contacted through the state office on aging.

About the Authors

VIRGINIA FRASER is currently the Long-Term Care Ombudsman for the State of Colorado. She was formerly on the faculty of Loretto Heights College in Denver.

SUSAN M. THORNTON is a writer and media consultant. Formerly a journalist with *U.S. News & World Report*, she has written about a wide range of topics for such publications as *The National Observer*, *Time* magazine, and *The Denver Post*.

www.ingramcontent.com/pod-product-compliance
Lightning Source LLC
Chambersburg PA
CBHW021119210326
41598CB00017B/1500